The Nurse's Dictionary:
500 Words Every Nurse Should Know

Minute Help Guides

Minute Help Press

www.minutehelpguides.com

© 2011

A

A&E [eɪ ənd iː] An abbreviation used in medicine to denote "accident and emergency".

A&W [eɪ ənd ˈdʌbljuː] A medical abbreviation used to describe a patient, meaning "alive and well".

a.c. [eɪ siː] An abbreviation for "ante cibum," meaning before meals. It is used as an instruction for administering medication.

A/O [eɪ əʊ] A medical abbreviation used to describe a patient, meaning "alert and oriented.

Abductor muscle [æbˈdʌktə(r) ˈmʌsl] Abductor muscles are those used to move a limb away from the midline of the body or adjacent body part, e.g. deltoid muscles for lifting the arm away from the body.

ABO blood group [eɪ biː əʊ blʌd gruːp] The major classification system for human blood. It is based on genetics and a person can be A, B, AB or O. The blood cell type affects the creation of antibodies, so blood of a different type may be rejected by the immune system during a transfusion.

Abortion [əˈbɔːʃn] The exit of a fetus from the uterus before it is viable. If it is spontaneous (not induced), it is termed a miscarriage.

ABP [eɪ biː piː] An abbreviation used for "arterial blood pressure"; which is the pressure exerted on the walls of an artery by the blood within it.

Abscess ['æbses] Any localized buildup of pus in the body. The pus accumulates in a cavity formed by the degradation of tissue by microorganisms.

ABW [eɪ biː 'dʌbljuː] An abbreviation used for "actual body weight," which is the measured weight of a patient.

Acquired immunity [əˈkwaɪə(r)d ɪˈmjuːnəti] Used in contrast to innate immunity, acquired immunity is developed during a life time from exposure to infection or vaccination.

Acquired [əˈkwaɪə(r)d] Something that is not innate but obtained during a life time. It is used to refer to immunity and diseases such as AIDS (Aquired Immunodeficiency Syndrome).

Activated charcoal ['æktɪveɪt 'tʃɑːkəʊl] Carbon that has been treated to increase its power of absorption by increasing its surface area (it is very porous). It has a number of applications including to bind poisons on swallowing.

Acute [əˈkjuːt] Occurring suddenly, progressing quickly and/or being of short duration. It is used to describe disease states in contrast to sub-acute and chronic.

ad lib [ˌæd 'lɪb] An abbreviation for "ad libitum," meaning use as much as desired. It is used as an instruction when prescribing a treatment or medication.

Adjuvant ['ædʒ ə vənt] An adjuvant is a substance that helps other substances to function, yet has little effect on its own. Adjuvants are used in vaccines to help elicit an immune reaction. Chemotherapy and radiation therapy for cancer are sometimes called adjuvant therapies.

ADR [eɪ diː ɑː(r)] A medical abbreviation to describe the negative effect of a pharmaceutical treatment on a patient, standing for "adverse drug reaction".

Adrenaline [əˈdrenəlɪn] Also known as epinephrine. Adrenaline is a hormone produced by the adrenal gland. It acts on the sympathetic nervous system, eliciting a flight or fight response.

Advanced practice nurse (APN) [ədˈvɑːnst ˈpræktɪs nɜːs] A nurse, also referred to as an advanced practice registered nurse (APRN), who has advanced education, skills and experience in a specialized field of nursing or in general.

Adverse reaction [ˈædvɜːs riˈækʃn] An undesired, dangerous and unexpected reaction to medication or treatment.

Afferent [ˈæf ər ənt] To carry towards a centre. It is used in contrast to efferent and can describe vessels and nerves in the body. Veins are afferent vessels as they carry blood towards the heart.

Afterbirth [ˈɑːftəbɜːθ] The expulsion of the placenta and fetal membranes through the birth canal after the birth of a baby. It usually occurs within an hour of childbirth and can be induced by the administration of oxytocin.

Aggressive [əˈgresɪv] Aggressive describes the manner in which some cancers or infections develop. Aggressive tumors are quick to grow and spread.

Airway [ˈeəweɪ] The pathway for air to enter the body to reach the lungs. Air enters through the nose or mouth, passes the pharynx and larynx and then goes through the trachea into the bronchi. It follows the same pathway to exit the body.

Akinesia [ˌeɪkɪˈniːsiə] A pathological inability to move due to a malfunction in the neuromuscular system. It is a common characteristic of advanced Parkinson's disease.

Alcoholism [ˈælkəhɒlɪzəm] An addiction to alcohol. It is characterized by excessive and compulsive consumption despite ill effects on own well-being and that of others. Chronic alcohol abuse can result in both physical and psychological dependencies as well as considerable tolerance to its effects.

Allergy scratch test [ˈælədʒi skrætʃ test] Also called a skin allergy test, it is a test done on the skin to detect allergic responses to different substances. A microscopic amount of a potential allergen is introduced onto a small scratch on the skin and the response is measured by assessing the resulting inflammation.

Allopathy [əˈlɒp ə θi] A type of medicine, also called conventional or western medicine. It was coined by the creator of homeopathy and is not always accepted by practitioners of conventional medicine.

Alopecia [ˌælə'piːʃə] Partial or complete hair loss or baldness. It can be pathological, the result of depilation, chemotherapy or it can be genetic (androgenic alopecia or male pattern balding in males and females).

Alternative medicine [ɔːl'tɜːnətɪv 'medɪsn] Alternative medicine is used to describe healing practices that do not fall into the normal methods of conventional, or western, medicine. It is usually not proven scientifically to be effective. It should not be confused with complementary medicine.

Amenorrhea [əˌmenə'riːə] The lack of menstruation in a woman of reproductive age. It can be pathological (often due to hormonal disturbances) or due to pregnancy, lactation or menopause.

Amniocentesis [ˌæmniəʊsen'tiːsɪs] The extraction of a small amount of amniotic fluid from the amnion, which contains fetal tissue. It is performed to test for genetic conditions and infections in the fetus. It is performed using a needle and carries some risk of miscarriage.

Amphetamine [æm'fetəmiːn] A psychoactive drug which promotes wakefulness and decreases appetite. Members of the amphetamine group of drugs are used to treat Attention deficit disorders and narcolepsy; however they are also commonly abused due to their performance boosting, appetite diminishing and euphoria inducing properties.

Ampule ['æmpuːl] A small sealed glass flask which typically contains injectable pharmaceutical chemicals and substances that react easily with air. It is opened by snapping off the top.

Analgesia [ˌænəlˈdʒiːziə] A lack of pain sensation whilst still conscious. Analgesics belong to a group of drugs that relieve pain.

Anaphylactic shock [ˌænəfɪˈlæktɪk ʃɒk] A severe and widespread acute allergic (hypersensitivity) reaction. It can be fatal and is characterized by low blood pressure and bronchoconstriction.

Anemia [əˈniːmiə] A state of having an abnormally low concentration of red blood cells or hemoglobin in the blood. This affects the efficiency with which the body can transport oxygen, leading to hypoxia.

Anesthesia [ˌænəsˈθiːʒə] A state of being without sensation. A local anesthetic blocks sensation in a localized area and a general anesthetic causes the recipient to temporarily lose consciousness. It allows for the administration of surgery or treatments that would otherwise cause considerable pain.

Aneurysm [ˈænjərɪzəm] An aneurysm is a localized ballooning of a blood vessel due to a weakening of the vessel wall. The "balloon" fills with blood and can rupture causing serious hemorrhaging and sometimes death. Aneurysms are common in the brain.

Antibody [ˈæntibɒdi] Also called immunoglobulins (Ig), antibodies are proteins that the immune system uses to identify and fight foreign substances or objects such as bacteria, viruses or pollen grains. The tips of antibodies bind antigens.

Antidote ['æntidəʊt] A substance that can counter the action of a poison, e.g. antivenom. Not all toxins have a known antidote.

Antiretroviral therapy (ART) [ˌænti ˌretrəʊ'vaɪrəl 'θerəpi] Medication given to fight infections by retroviruses such as HIV. It sometimes includes a number of drugs given in combination. (HAART-highly active ART).

Antiseptic [ˌænti'septɪk] An antiseptic is a substance that is antimicrobial; able to kill bacteria and viruses. Used in contrast to antibacterial (can limit bacterial growth, not necessarily kill them) and disinfectant (for use on non-living objects only).

Apgar score ['æp gɑr skɔː(r)] A score used to measure the health of a baby immediately after being born. The score is out of 10 and assesses the "Appearance, Pulse, Grimace, Activity and Respiration" of the infant. The test is normally done one and five minutes after birth and repeated if the score remains low.

Apnea [æp'niːə] Apnea is a state of suspended breathing. Breathing can be suspended voluntarily, by a mechanical force, as the result of disease or it can be drug induced. Sleep apnea is a condition where breathing stops whilst sleeping, causing the sufferer to wake to restart respiration.

Appendix [ə'pendɪks] The appendix is a blind-ended, worm shaped, vestigial organ situated near the junction of the small and large intestine. It has no real function but can become inflamed and require removal.

Arrhythmia [əˈrɪð mi ə] Arrhythmia is also called Cardiac dysrhythmia. It refers to a group of conditions characterized by abnormal electrical impulses in the heart, which cause an irregular heart rate. It can result in cardiac arrest.

Arthritis [ɑːˈθraɪtɪs] A broad term to describe conditions affecting the joints in the body. The most common include osteoarthritis and rheumatoid arthritis. It is associated with considerable pain, reduced function and physical deformation.

Aspirin [ˈæsprɪn] Also called acetylsalicylic acid, aspirin is a very common drug used as an anti-inflammatory, an analgesic and an antipyretic, as well as an anti-platelet agent in people prone to thrombosis. It is the major non-steroidal anti-inflammatory drug.

Assay [əˈseɪ] A test of the activity or amount of a substance. There are many types of assays that can be performed including immunoassays, enzymatic activity assays and cell viability assays.

Asthma [ˈæsmə] Asthma is a chronic inflammatory disease of the airways, which affects breathing and manifests as coughing, wheezing and struggling to breathe. It can be caused by allergens and is usually characterized by acute asthma attacks. It can be treated by inhaling corticosteroids.

Asymptomatic [ˌeɪsɪmptəˈmætɪk] Showing no symptoms. Asymptomatic is used to describe a patient who carries a disease or infection but shows no symptoms normally associated with the disease. Symptoms can sometimes arise later or the disease can resolve itself with symptoms never arising. Also referred to as sub-clinical infection.

Ateriosclerosis [ɑːˌtɪəriəʊskləˈrəʊsɪs] The buildup of fatty substances, especially cholesterol, in the arteries. It is the major cause of heart disease as the plaques can block the flow of blood to and/or from the heart. It is also called the hardening of arteries.

Atopic [eɪˈtɒpɪk] Atopy is an allergic reaction in parts of the body that are not necessarily in contact with the allergen. It is generally used for a genetic predisposition to hypersensitivity reactions.

Attenuated vaccine [əˈtenjueɪtɪd ˈvæksiːn] An attenuated vaccine is one that uses a living pathogen with decreased virulence e.g. the measles, chicken pox and yellow fever vaccines. Used in contrast to an inactivated vaccine where the infectious agent is killed.

Autoimmune [ˌɔːtəʊɪˈmjuːn] Autoimmunity is when the immune system recognizes the body's own cells as foreign and mounts an immune response. It is a failure of the immune system to recognize "self" cells.

Autopsy [ˈɔːtɒpsi] A medical procedure undertaken after death to determine the cause of death or to identify any other abnormality. It is also called a post-mortem.

B

b.i.d. (or BID) [biː aɪ diː] Latin for "bis in die" meaning twice in a day, normally used as an instruction for administering prescribed medicine.

Basal metabolic rate ['beɪsl ˌmetə'bɒlɪk reɪt] The basal metabolic rate is the underlying, or resting rate of energy expenditure. This is usually measured after fasting and while at rest.

Bed sore ['bedsɔː(r)] A lesion caused most frequently by pressure and exacerbated by urine, micro-organisms, medication and age. They occur predominantly in bed-ridden patients who are not moved often enough.

Benign [bɪ'naɪn] The term benign is usually used to describe tumors that are not cancerous or malignant. It is not invasive (spreading into other tissue) but does grow in situ.

Bile [baɪl] Bile is a liquid substance produced by the liver and stored in the gallbladder. It acts in the duodenum via the common bile duct to aid digestion.

Bilirubin [ˌbɪlɪ'ruːbɪn] One of the products in the breakdown of hemoglobin in red blood cells. It is yellow/orange in color.

Biopsy ['baɪɒpsi] Generally used for making diagnoses, a biopsy is the removal of a small amount of tissue for visualization of the cells, usually under a microscope.

Blood clot [blʌd klɒt] Also called a thrombus; a blood clot is an aggregation of platelets through the process of coagulation. It occurs normally through injury or pathologically as a thrombosis.

Blood count [blʌd kaʊnt] A full or complete blood count measures the number of red bloods cells (erythrocytes), white blood cells (leukocytes) and platelets (thrombocytes) in a unit of blood. Abnormalities in the count can indicate disease states.

Blood plasma [blʌd ˈplæzmə] Blood plasma is the liquid part of blood in which the blood cells are suspended. It is made predominantly of water and dissolved proteins and sugars as well as minerals, clotting factors and carbon dioxide.

Blood pressure [blʌd ˈpreʃə(r)] Blood pressure is a measure of the pressure of circulating blood on the walls of blood vessels. It is one of the vital signs. It is measured as the systolic pressure (maximum) over diastolic pressure (minimum), averaged over a number of heart beats.

Blood transfusion [blʌd trænsˈfjuːʒn] A medical procedure of transferring blood or components of blood from a donor to a patient. It is a lifesaving technique used when there is major blood loss, during trauma or surgery, or in the case of severe anemia. It is associated with some risk of transferring blood parasites and infections as well as if blood of a different type is used.

Body mass index: ['bɒdi mæs 'ɪndeks] An index used to assess the relationship between a person's height and weight. It is defined as weight in kilograms (kg) divided by height in meters (m) squared. Mid-range values indicate a healthy weight in relation to height.

Bone mineral density [bəʊn 'mɪnərəl 'densəti] Bone mineral density (BMD) is a measure of the density of bones (how much matter there is per unit squared). Low values can indicate the presence of or a susceptibility to osteoporosis.

Botulism ['bɒtjulɪzəm] A rare but serious disease caused by the bacterium Clostridium botulinum. It produces a toxin that causes nerve paralysis and which is used cosmetically as "botox".

Bradycardia [ˌbræd ɪ'kɑr di ə] Bradycardia is a resting heart rate lower than 60 beats per minute. Cardiac arrest can occur if it drops below 50 beats per minute.

Braxton Hicks contractions ['bræk'stəʊn hɪks kən'trækʃn] The "practice" contractions of the uterus that occur near the end of pregnancy. They are differentiated from true labor contractions by their irregularity.

Bypass ['baɪpɑːs] A surgical method of creating an alternative passage for fluids or substances to pass. Common bypass surgeries include the gastric bypass and coronary artery bypass.

C

Caesarian section [sɪˈzeərɪən ˈsekʃn] A surgical procedure to deliver a baby or dead fetus. It involves making an incision through the abdomen and uterus of the mother. It is normally indicated if the baby is in distress, if normal labor does not progress or if the baby is laying breech.

Capillary [kəˈpɪləri] A capillary is the smallest type of blood vessel found in the microcirculation system. It allows for the exchange of gases and nutrients between the blood and tissue at a cellular level. They arise from arterioles and venules.

Carcinogen [kɑːˈsɪnədʒən] A carcinogen is substance that directly promotes the development of cancer. It includes radiation and toxins. They normally act by damaging the DNA of cells, causing mutations that result in unchecked cell growth.

Carcinoma [ˌkɑːsɪˈnəʊmə] A carcinoma is a malignant tumor originating from epithelial, or similar, cells.

Case Management [keɪs ˈmænɪdʒmənt] The coordination of long term patient care by a case manager, especially for patients with chronic conditions.

Catatonia [ˌkætəˈtəʊnɪə] A state associated with psychological and motor disturbance, characterized by a loss of movement or repetitive movement, often holding the same pose for extended periods. It can occur with schizophrenia, bipolar disorder, major depression, some infections and from drug induction or withdrawal.

Catheter ['kæθɪtə(r)] A tube that is inserted into a body cavity, vessel or duct. It is used to drain fluids from the bladder or sites of infection and can be left inserted for a period of time or even permanently. It can also be used to administer substances into the body.

Cauterization ['kɔːtəraɪzeɪʃn] A method of burning part of the body to seal it by killing some tissue. It is used less often now but historically has been used to stop bleeding at sites of severe injury, closing amputation sites and sterilizing sites of infection.

CD 4 [ˌsiː ˈdiː fɔː(r)] CD 4 stands for Cluster of Differentiation 4. It is a glycoprotein found at the surface of a number of immune system cells (T-cells, monocytes, dendritic cells, macrophages). A CD 4 count is done to estimate the function of the immune system, especially in people with AIDS.

Certified nurse-midwife (CNM) ['sɜːtɪfaɪd nɜːs 'mɪdwaɪf] A registered nurse with some advanced education in the field of maternity nursing, usually a master's degree that can be through the American College of Nurse-Midwives.

Certified registered nurse anesthetist (CRNA) ['sɜːtɪfaɪd 'redʒɪstə(r)d nɜːs ə'niːsθətɪst] An advanced practice registered nurse who has additional training recognized by the American Association of Nurse Anesthetists, in the administration of anesthetics.

Cervix ['sɜːvɪks] The cervix is the neck of the uterus; a narrowing where the uterus joins the vagina. Part of the cervix is visible using a speculum.

Chemotherapy [ˌkiːməʊˈθerəpi] Technically, chemotherapy is the treatment of illness with chemicals, however it more often refers to the chemical treatment of cancer with antineoplastic drugs.

Cholesterol [kəˈlestərɒl] Cholesterol is an important component of cell membranes to maintain balance in its fluidity. It is a sterol made mostly in animals. Excessive cholesterol intake can increase the risk of heart disease.

Chronic ['krɒnɪk] On-going or lasting a long time. A chronic condition is normally one that last longer than three months. It is in contrast to "acute".

Circulating nurse ['sɜːkjəleɪtɪŋ nɜːs] A surgical nurse who circulates the operating room to ensure that the procedure is done in sterile conditions and monitors the progress of the surgery, sometimes with administrative responsibilities.

Cleft palate [kleft ˈpælət] A congenital deformity that can occur alone or together with a cleft lip. It results from abnormal facial development during embryogenesis. It can be treated surgically.

Clinical Nurse Leader (CNL) ['klɪnɪkl nɜːs ˈliːdə(r)] A clinical nurse leader is a registered nurse with advanced education in clinical nursing with a specific focus on leadership and skills training in health care facilities. CNLs are certified by the Commission on Nurse Certivication.

Clinical nurse specialist (CNS) [ˈklɪnɪkl nɜːs ˈspeʃəlɪst] An advanced practice nurse who has advanced education (normally a master's degree) in the specialized field of clinical science, which is concerned with administering evidence-based therapies.

Clinical trial [ˈklɪnɪkl ˈtraɪəl] Trials which assess the safety and efficacy of medical treatments on humans once non-clinical data has indicated that it is safe for human application.

Cochlear implant [ˈkɒkliə(r) ɪmˈplɑːnt] A surgically implanted prosthetic in the ear to provide a sense of hearing to the deaf or profoundly hard of hearing.

Colostomy bag [kəˈlɒstəmi bæg] Also called an ostomy pouching system, it is a bag that collects waste diverted from the colon, ileum or bladder.

Coma [ˈkəʊmə] The state of unconsciousness lasting an extended period of time and from which a person cannot be roused. There is no response to stimuli and waking from a coma is spontaneous and unexplained.

Co-morbid [koʊˈmɔːbɪd] The occurrence of one or more disease or disorder together. Some conditions commonly occur co-morbidly, such as AIDS and Tuberculosis or ADHD and bipolar disorder.

Complication [ˌkɒmplɪˈkeɪʃn] A medical complication is an undesired and unplanned negative occurrence associated with a disease or treatment. In the case of disease it can become worse or have additional symptoms. Complications can be iatrogenic.

Computed tomography [kəmˈpjuːtɪd təˈmɒgrəfi] Also called a CT scan, computed tomography is a method of medical imaging that uses X-rays and digital computing to obtain three dimensional images of internal objects.

Concussion [kənˈkʌʃn] A concussion is a minor trauma to the head. The term is used more commonly in sports medicine and MTBI (Mild Traumatic Brain Injury) preferred in medicine generally. Symptoms can be physical, emotional and cognitive depending on the nature of the concussion.

Congenital [kənˈdʒenɪtl] Normally referring to a disease, congenital conditions are those which are hereditary or which occur during the baby's development in utero.

Contusion [kənˈtjuːʒn] A contusion is an area of hemorrhage under the skin as a result of mechanical damage. Contusions are also called bruises.

Cortisone [ˈkɔːtɪzəʊn] Cortisone is a steroid hormone used to treat a variety of conditions. It suppresses the immune system and so is used to treat inflammation and autoimmune disorders, however its long-term usage carries some health risks.

Critical Care ['krɪtɪkl keə(r)] A type of medical intervention and facility for patients who are critically ill or injured.

Critical care nursing ['krɪtɪkl keə(r) 'nɜːsɪŋ] The field of nursing that deals with patients in a critical state, usually in intensive care units of hospitals and emergency rooms.

Cruciate ligament ['kru ʃi ɪt 'lɪgəmənt] Cruciate ligaments are configured in the shape of an "X" and are found in pairs in a number of joints of the body, including the knee. They provide stability whilst allowing for movement.

Cyst [sɪst] A closed sac that contains gas or fluids. A membrane separates it from surrounding tissue. It should not be confused with an abscess. Some cysts need to be removed surgically.

D

Defibrillation [ˌdiːfɪbrɪˈleɪʃn] Defibrillation is a
method of treating heart failure using a defibrillator
which sends electrical impulses to the heart and so
restarting the sinoatrial node to act as pacemaker.

Dialysis [ˌdaɪˈæləsɪs] Primarily a treatment for
patients who have lost the function of their kidneys,
dialysis artificially replaces the function of the
kidneys by filtering the blood.

Diastole [daɪˈæstəli] The time after systole when the
heart fills with blood. The heart muscle is relaxed
during diastole and alternates between the atria and
ventricles so that blood is pushed through the heart.
In the arteries it refers to the lowest pressure exerted
on the vessel walls.

Diazepam [daɪˈæzəpæm] A benzodiazepine drug
first marketed as Valium. It is a central nervous
system depressant used for the treatment of anxiety,
insomnia and some seizures, as well as being used
recreationally.

Differential diagnosis [ˌdɪfəˈrenʃl ˌdaɪəgˈnəʊsɪs]
When more than one disease fits a set of symptoms,
a differential diagnosis is made to compare clinical
signs and eliminate possible diagnoses until the true
one is identified.

Dilation [daɪˈleɪʃn] To dilate means to enlarge or
expand and in medicine usually refers to blood
vessels, the cervix and the pupil in the eye. It is
used in contrast to contraction.

Diuretic [ˌdaɪjuˈretɪk] A substance that increases the rate of urine excretion.

Do not resuscitate order [də nɒt rɪˈsʌsɪteɪt ˈɔːdə(r)] Also called a Living Will. It is a binding legal document signed when healthy and of sound mind that states that attempts at resuscitation should not be undertaken if the person experiences cardiac or respiratory failure.

Doctor assisted suicide [ˈdɒktə(r) əˈsɪstɪd ˈsuːɪsaɪd] In medicine, assisted suicide normally refers to helping a terminally ill person who wants to die to end their life by either providing the means for them to kill themselves or by administering the means. It is highly controversial and in most countries, illegal.

Dopamine [ˈdəʊpəmiːn] A catecholamine neurotransmitter produced in the brain. It has various functions in behavior, reward, cognition and prolactin production.

Douche [duːʃ] The rinsing of a body cavity using a stream of water. It usually refers to vaginal irrigation.

Drug resistance [drʌg rɪˈzɪstəns] The reduced efficacy of a drug to treat a disease; mostly used to describe the failure of antibiotic treatment to kill the target microbe. Resistance is an acquired state achieved by natural selection. Multi and extreme drug resistance occurs when microbes are resistant to more than one antibiotic drug.

DSM-IV [di: es em fɔ:(r)] The Diagnostic and Statistical Manual of Mental Disorders is a set of standardized terms and criteria for diagnoses published by the American Psychiatric Association and used in many countries.

Dysentery ['dɪsəntri] A disease characterized by inflammation of the colon, normally caused by bacterial, viral or amebic infection. The stool is watery and can contain blood. It results in fever and dehydration, and if left untreated, death.

Dysphoria [dɪs'fɔ:riə] A depressed mood, used in contrast to euphoria. It can refer to low moods in healthy people or be a symptom of a more serious mental illness; depression is characterized by extended periods of dysphoria.

Dystonia [dɪs'toʊ ni ə] A movement disorder that results in abnormal muscle contraction. It produces repetitive and twisting motions in particular.

E

Eclampsia [ɪˈklæmpsɪə] Convulsions in patients
with preeclampsia that are not due to epilepsy or
other brain damage.

Edema [ɪˈdiːmə] Previously known as dropsy,
edema is the abnormal accumulation of fluid in cells
or between cells and the consequent visual swelling
of affected areas. Edema can be fatal as in the case
of pulmonary edema.

Efferent [ˈɛf ər ənt] To carry away from a centre;
efferent can be used to describe blood vessels which
carry blood away from the heart (arteries), or nerves
which conduct signals away from the central
nervous system. It is the opposite of afferent.

Electrocardiogram (ECG, EKG)
[ɪˌlektrəʊˈkɑːdiəʊɡræm] A measurement and
graphic representation of the heart's electrical
activity as voltage over time. It is a non-invasive
means to evaluate the functioning of the heart.

Electroencephalogram (EEG)
[ɪˌlektrəʊɪnˈsefələɡræm] The measurement and
graphical representation of the electrical activity of
the neurons in the brain. It is used in the diagnosis
of strokes, comas and other brain disorders.

Emaciation [ɪˌmeɪsiˈeɪʃn] The process of becoming
very thin from the loss of body mass. It can be a
result of disease or malnutrition.

Embolism ['embəlɪzəm] The blockage or occlusion of a vessel by an embolus, which can be gas or solid.

Emergency Nursing [iˈmɜːdʒənsi ˈnɜːsɪŋ] The field of nursing that deals with patients in need of emergency care, often when critically ill or injured. The care is normally required before a diagnosis of the disease or injury has been made. Such nurses are termed Certified Emergency Nurse (in the USA).

Endemic [enˈdemɪk] Used in epidemiology, endemic refers to a pattern of disease occurrence that is relatively stable in its frequency over time.

Endocrine [ˈendəʊkrɪn] Endocrine refers to the glands and gland secretions of ductless hormonal glands internally. It is used in contrast to exocrine.

Endogenous [enˈdɒdʒənəs] A substance, process or condition that originates from within the body, its tissue or cells.

Endoscope [ˈendəskəʊp] An instrument that allows for the observation of the interior of organs and body cavities. It usually consists of a small camera and light at the end of a tube structure.

Enema [ˈenəmə] A procedure for clearing out the bowel by injecting fluids into the rectum. It is indicated in severe cases of constipation or for the administration of medication.

Enteritis [ˌentəˈraɪtəs] Enteritis is the inflammation of the small intestine, normally resulting from infection by pathogenic microbes. It is characterized by abdominal pain, diarrhea and fever.

Epidemiology [ˌepɪˌdiːmiˈɒlədʒi] The study of the distribution of disease and health condition occurrences at a population level. It is important for the understanding of how infectious diseases emerge and in the management of public health.

Epidural [ˌepɪˈdjʊərəl] Epidural means on or outside one of the spinal cord membranes called the dura mater. It is also used to refer to a type of regional anesthetic which causes a loss of sensation from the waist down, which is injected into the epidural space outside the dura mater. This anesthetic is commonly used for childbirth.

Epilepsy [ˈepɪlepsi] A chronic neurological disorder resulting from episodic abnormal neural discharge. This causes seizures that vary greatly in form. Epilepsy can be controlled by medication.

Episiotomy [ɪˌpiːsiˈɒtəmi] A surgical procedure that involves cutting the base of the vulva. It is usually performed to avoid tearing of the skin of vulva during childbirth but can also be to aid vaginal surgery.

Epistaxis [ˌep əˈstæk sɪs] More commonly known as a nosebleed, epistaxis is the loss of blood from the nose through the nostril. Causes include blunt trauma, foreign bodies, allergic response and infections.

Erythema [ˌɛr ə'θi mə] A reddening due to vasodilation which normally indicates a site of infection or inflammation.

Etiology [ˌiːti'ɒlədʒi] The study of origins or causes. In medicine it is usually used to describe the cause of disease.

Exacerbation [ɪg'zæsəbeɪt] An increase in the severity of a disease or of its symptoms. It is the worsening or making worse of a disease state.

Excision [ɪk'sɪʒn] The surgical removal or cutting out of a structure or part of a structure. In molecular biology it refers to a process whereby genetic material is cut out of the DNA.

Exocrine ['eksəʊkraɪn] Exocrine refers to the glands and gland secretions of ducted glands. It is used in contrast to endocrine.

Exogenous [ek'sɒdʒənəs] Exogenous describes substances or processes that do not originate inside the organism. Used in contrast to endogenous.

Extensor [ɪk'stensə(r)] A type of muscle which, on contraction, causes a body part to become more straight such that the parts which are proximal and distal to the joint become further apart. An extensor antagonizes a flexor.

Extraction [ɪk'strækʃn] In dentistry an extraction is the surgical removal of a tooth from the alveolus. In medicine it can refer to the removal of something by pulling it out.

Failure to thrive [ˈfeɪljə(r) tuː θraɪv] A phrase used to describe a condition in infants when they fail to gain weight or do not grow at the normal rate. It can be caused by something congenital or by malnourishment.

F

Familial [fəˈmɪliəl] A condition that occurs more frequently in related people than can be considered by chance. It is normally used to describe genetic conditions.

Febrile [ˈfiːbraɪl] Febrile refers to or is related to fever (pyrexia), which is characterized by high body temperatures.

Ferritin [ˈferɪtɪn] A protein found in the body which stores iron and releases it when necessary, providing protection from anemia.

Fetal alcohol syndrome [ˈfiːtl ˈælkəhɒl ˈsɪndrəʊm] A condition resulting from excessive alcohol consumption during pregnancy. It is characterized by malformation, especially cranio-facial, and mental retardation in the baby.

Fever [ˈfiːvə(r)] High core body temperature in response to disease, also called pyrexia. It is a medical sign of infection and is accompanied by the activation of the immune system.

Fibrosis [faɪˈbrəʊsɪs] The formation of fibrous tissue, which is not a natural part of the body. It can be part of tissue repair (scarring) or in reaction to something, such as in cirrhosis.

First degree burn [fɜːst dɪˈgriː bɜːn] An injury to the exterior of the body caused by heat (from friction, radiation, chemical, fire etc.). Also called a superficial burn, it only involves damage to the epidermis. It is used in contrast to second and third degree burns.

Flaccid ['flæsɪd] Lacking tone; normally used to describe a type of paralysis where there is a complete or partial loss of muscle tone in part or all of the body.

Folic acid [ˌfɒlɪk ˈæsɪd] Folic acid and folate are forms of vitamin B9. It is important for the manufacture of DNA. Deficiencies are associated with neurological defects such as anemia. In utero, deficiencies can result in fatal conditions like spina bifida.

Food and Drug Administration (FDA) [fuːd ənd drʌg ədˌmɪnɪˈstreɪʃn] A regulating body of the Department of Health and Human Services in the United States. They protect public health by controlling the safety of food and pharmaceuticals in the country.

Forceps ['fɔːseps] Forceps are an instrument for grasping and holding objects. It is handheld and used when the fingers are inadequate for reaching or gripping objects or tissue.

Forceps delivery ['fɔːseps dɪˈlɪvəri] A childbirth that is aided by the use of forceps, which grasp the head of the fetus whilst still in the birth canal and help pull it out. It is associated with some risk of injury to the fetus and mother but is indicated when the fetus fails to progress down the birth canal and becomes distressed.

Foreign body ['fɒrən 'bɒdi] A substance or object in the tissue or body cavities that is exogenous; originating from outside the body. It is typically something that the body cannot readily absorb.

Fracture ['fræktʃə(r)] A break in a bone from the application of stress. There are many different types of fracture, including simple (a clean break across the bone) compound (where the skin is broken and the break exposed), incomplete (where the break is partial) and fissured (cracks in the bone, especially of the cranium and face).

Frontal ['frʌntl] An anatomical term of location referring to the anterior part of the body or the frontal plane.

Fulminating ['fʊlmɪneɪtɪŋ] A term describing a disease that runs its course quickly or deteriorates quickly.

G

Gangrene [ˈgæŋgriːn] Gangrene is the death of tissue due to a loss or decrease in blood supply. It can affect an extremity or organ.

General [ˈdʒenrəl] General refers to something that occurs all over the body, not in one specific area. It is used in contrast to regional and local.

Gerontology [ˌdʒerɒnˈtɒlədʒi] The study of aging and diseases that are typically associated with geriatrics, or the aged.

Gingivitis [ˌdʒɪndʒɪˈvaɪtəs] Inflammation of the gums or gingiva, normally as a result of bacterial infection. It presents as reddening with edema and sometimes bleeding.

Glaucoma [glɔːˈkəʊmə] An eye disease resulting from inadequate drainage of interocular fluids through the trabecular meshwork. The increased pressure can damage the optic nerve, which results in partial or complete blindness if not treated.

Glucagon [ˈgluːkəˌgɒn] A hormone secreted by the pancreas that has the opposite action of insulin, that is, it raises the blood sugar levels by causing the conversion of glycogen to glucose by the liver.

Glycogen [ˈglaɪkədʒən] Glycogen a molecule that acts as a glucose store in the liver. It is converted to glucose on secretion of glucagon. It is similar to starch in structure and character.

Goiter ['gɔɪtə(r)] A chronic condition characterized by an enlarged thyroid gland, the most common cause of which being a deficiency in iodine which is necessary for proper thyroid function.

Graft [grɑːft] A transplantation of tissue or organ. Often used to describe a skin graft where skin from one part of the body is transplanted to another to repair damage such as that caused by third degree burns.

Gram stain [græm steɪn] A type of differential stain for bacteria to distinguish between types with a thick peptidoglycan wall (gram-positive) and those without (gram-negative). The two types of bacteria also have other differences, which can be important when treating bacterial infections.

H

Habitus ['hæbɪtɪs] A person's physique or physical
characteristics including appearance and
susceptibility to disease.

Hallucination [hə‚luːsɪˈneɪʃn] A subjective
perception of external stimuli which does not exist
in reality. It can affect any of the senses and can
result from psychosis, drug use, falling into and
waking from sleep, sleep deprivation and
neurological disorders.

Head nurse [hed nɜːs] The nurse, also called a
charge nurse, who is responsible for the functioning
and administration of a hospital unit, usually on a
shift basis.

Heart massage [hɑːt ˈmæsɑːʒ] Also called
Cardiopulmonary resuscitation (CPR), it is the
massage or squeezing of the heart through the chest
or through an open chest in order to imitate the
heart's action to circulate the blood during
resuscitation after cardiac arrest.

Heatstroke [ˈhiːtstrəʊk] A serious condition
resulting from exposure to excessive temperatures
especially in addition to exertion. It can be fatal and
is characterized by dehydration, vertigo, confusion
and if severe, coma.

Hematocrit [hɪˈmæt ə krɪt] Hematocrit or packed
cell volume is the proportion of cells in a unit of

blood. Abnormal hematocrit levels can indicate the presence of disease.

Hematology [ˌhiːməˈtɒlədʒi] The study of blood and the tissue that forms it, including its structure, function, pathology and therapy. A physician that specialises in haematology is a haematologist.

Hemoglobin [ˌhiːməˈgləʊbɪn] Hemoglobin is an iron containing protein found in red blood cells. It gives erythrocytes their red color. It can bind oxygen for distribution through the body.

Hemorrhage [ˈhemərɪdʒ] Also referred to as bleeding, it is the escape of blood from the vessels into surrounding tissue or out of the body.

Hemorrhoids [ˈhemərɔɪdz] Hemorrhoids normally refers to a phathological varicose vein of the hemorrhoid vessels in the anus. It results in painful swelling and inflammation. Can also be called piles.

Hepatitis [ˌhepəˈtaɪtɪs] The inflammation of the liver, most often as the result of infection by one of the hepatitis viruses which cause Hepatitis A, B, C, D and E, or by the Epstein-Barr Virus, Yellow fever or Herpes simplex. Non-viral causes of hepatitis include toxoplasma and Leptospira.

Hereditary [həˈredɪtri] A condition is considered hereditary if it is passed down or is able to be passed down from parent to child by the genes. It can refer to physical characters like eye color or diseases such as hemophilia.

Hermetic [hɜːˈmetɪk] Airtight, normally referring to vessels or containers that are sealed to exclude air.

Hernia [ˈhɜːniə] A protrusion of an organ or tissue through the wall of tissue that normally contains it. It is common in the abdomen from weak spots in the muscular abdominal wall.

Hippocampus [ˌhɪpəˈkæmpəs] The hippocampus is a part of the brain that is part of the limbic system. It is important for long-term memory and special orientation. It has a paired structure and is housed in the medial temporal lobe of the brain.

Hippocratic Oath [ˌhɪpəkrætɪk ˈəʊθ] The oath taken by medical doctors when they qualify for a doctoral degree. It is a promise to honor a number of ethical rules which it outlines.

Histocompatibility [hɪˈstɒkəmˌpætəˈbɪləti] Identity or similarity in the immune system, which is required for successful tissue or organ transplants.

Hodgkin's lymphoma [ˈhɒdʒkɪnz lɪmˈfəʊmə] A cancer originating from lymphocytes. The lymphoma spreads from one lymph node to another and the primary symptom is enlargement of the lymph nodes and frequently the spleen and liver as well.

Home health nurse [həʊm helθ nɜːs] Also called a visiting nurse; this is a nurse who works with a client or group of clients in their own homes.

Homeopathy [ˌhəʊmiˈɒpəθi] A type of alternative therapy based on a theory of "like cures like".

Treatments are typically highly diluted or of very small dose. Homeopathy is not evidence based and not recognized in conventional medicine. It is thought to be only as effective as the placebo effect.

Hospital Emergency Code ['hɒspɪtl i'mɜ:dʒənsi kəʊd] These codes are used in hospitals to alert staff of types of emergency situations. They are normally color based (code red, code blue etc.) but their use is not standardized or universal.

Hydropenia ['haɪ droʊ'pi ni ə] More commonly referred to as dehydration, hydropenia is a deficiency in body fluids resulting from a loss of water, loss of electrolytes or the loss of both.

Hymen ['haɪmən] A thin membrane that partly covers the vaginal ostium prior to its rupture. It is not always present but is often used as an indication of virginity.

Hypercalcemia [ˌhaɪ pər kæl'si mi ə] A state of having abnormally high concentrations of calcium ions in the blood which presents with a set of symptoms (including constipation and lethargy) and can indicate disease.

Hyperglycemia [ˌhaɪpəglaɪ'si:miə] A state of having an abnormally high level of glucose in the blood. Especially found in diabetic patients.

Hyperplasia [ˌhaɪ pər'pleɪ ʒə] An increased number of cells as a normal response to a stimulus and not normally attributable to neoplasia.

Hyperpnea [ˌhaɪ pərp'ni ə] An increased rate and depth of breathing as compared to that at rest.

Hypersensitivity [ˌhaɪpəˌsensə'tɪvəti] A heightened sensitivity to a stimulus, used especially in reference to an immune system that reacts with undesired effects.

Hypertension (HTN) [ˌhaɪpə'tenʃn] Abnormally high blood pressure which can be transient or sustained. It occurs when the systolic blood pressure (when the heart contracts) is over 140 mmHg and/or the diastolic (when the heart is relaxed) is above 90 mmHg. It is associated with a risk of cardiovascular damage.

Hypocalcemia [ˌhaɪ poʊ kæl'si mi ə] A state of having abnormally low concentrations of calcium ions in the blood, normally due to a deficiency in parathyroid hormone (PTH) from a number of causes.

Hypocapnia ['haɪpəʊkæpnɪə] The state of having abnormally low levels of carbon dioxide in the blood. It can be caused by excessive breathing (hyperventilation).

Hypodermic needle [ˌhaɪpə'dɜːmɪk 'niːdl] A hollow needle used in conjunction with a syringe to inject or extract liquid substances just below the skin.

Hypoglycemia [ˌhaɪpəʊglaɪ'siːmɪə] A state of having an abnormally low level of glucose in the blood. Symptoms can include trembling, nausea and sweating, confusion and tiredness.

Hypotension [ˈhaɪpəʊˈtenʃn] Abnormally low blood pressure, which can be transient or sustained. It occurs when the systolic blood pressure (when the heart contracts) is less than 90mmHg and/or the diastolic (when the heart is relaxed) is below 60mmHg.

I

Iatric [aɪˈæ trɪk] Relating to medicine or a medical doctor or healer, as in iatrogenic; an effect caused by a medical practitioner.

Iatrogenic [aɪˌæ trəˈdʒɛn ɪk] Inadvertently caused by a health care professional. It refers to adverse reactions and complications that result from a treatment, drug or advice given.

Ibuprofen [ˌaɪbjuːˈprəʊfen] A commonly used non-steroidal anti-inflammatory and analgesic when pain is associated with inflammation. Ibuprofen is derived from propionic acid. Its anti-platelet effect is much less than that of aspirin.

ICD code [ˌaɪ siː diː kəʊd] ICD is the International Classification of Diseases from the World Health Organization. It uses a system of alphanumerical codes to standardize the description of medical conditions.

Idiopathic [ˌɪdiəˈpæθɪk] A term used to describe a condition that has no known cause.

in situ [ˌɪn ˈsɪtjuː] A Latin term meaning "in position", especially used to describe something that has not moved since its origin. To view something in situ is to see it where it normally occurs. In oncology a tumor in situ is one that has not invaded other tissue.

in utero [ˌɪn ˈjuːtərəʊ] A Latin term meaning "in the uterus" or not yet born in reference to a fetus.

in vitro [ɪn ˈviːtrəʊ] A Latin term referring to an artificial environment, normally in a test tube or other medium in a laboratory.

in vitro fertilization (IVF) [ɪn ˈviːtrəʊ ˌfɜːtəlaɪˈzeɪʃn] The process of achieving fertilization in a culture medium in a laboratory and then introducing the resulting zygote into the uterus to implant and develop into a fetus.

in vivo [ɪn ˈviːvəʊ] Inside a living organism, can be plant or animal. Normally used in contrast to "in vitro" (meaning in the laboratory).

Incontinence [ɪnˈkɒntɪnəns] The involuntary excretion of urine or feces due to an inability to control the bowels or bladder. It is normally treatable and caused by an underlying medical condition.

Infarction [ɪnˈfɑːkʃn] An area of tissue death, or necrosis, resulting from a lack of oxygen to the cells. It can be caused by a blockage in the supply of oxygenated blood that is pathological, mechanical or drug induced in origin.

Infectious [ɪnˈfekʃəs] Infectious refers to a disease, normally caused by a microorganism, which can be passed between people with or without contact.

Inferior [ɪnˈfɪəriə(r)] An anatomical term of location, especially in human anatomy, meaning towards the feet or below; similar to posterior. It is used in contrast to superior.

Inflammation [ˌɪnfləˈmeɪʃn] A complex response of the vascular system to infection, irritation or injury. It presents a swelling and reddening as there is increased blood flow to the affected area as well as an influx of immune cells.

Inflammatory bowel disease (IBD) [ɪnˈflæmətri ˈbaʊəl dɪˈziːz] A chronic condition affecting the intestines resulting in inflammation. The primary types of IBD are Crohn's disease and ulcerative colitis.

Infusion Therapy [ɪnˈfjuːʒn ˈθerəpi] Administration of fluids, including medicine, intravenously through a drip.

Inoculate [ɪˈnɒkjuleɪt] The process of introducing a substance into the body to boost the immunity to it, such as in the case of vaccination. It also refers to the substance that is introduced.

Insulin [ˈɪnsjəlɪn] A hormone that is secreted by the pancreas in response to high sugar levels and which promotes the conversion of glucose into glycogen.

int. cib. [ɪnˈtɜː(r) si bɔs] An abbreviation for the Latin term "inter cibos" meaning between meals.

Intensive care unit (ICU) [ɪnˈtensɪv keə(r) ˈjuːnɪt] A hospital facility that provides a high level and intensity of medical care for critically ill patients. It involves continuous monitoring and nursing and the availability of equipment for resuscitating patients.

Interaction [ˌɪntərˈækʃn] In pharmacology, a drug interaction is the combined effect of two or more drugs in the body, which can be different from the individual effect of each drug independently.

Intern [ɪnˈtɜːn] A final year student or graduate who gains practical experience in medicine by working under the supervision of a medical professional in a hospital and in the unit of their chosen field.

Intrauterine device (IUD) [ˌɪntrəˈjuːtəraɪn dɪˈvaɪs] A contraceptive device that is inserted in the uterus. It can be made of copper-containing substances or it can release progesterone and comes in a variety of shapes.

Intravenous (IV, I.V., i.v.) [ˌɪntrəˈviːnəs] Intravenous means within a vein. It is normally used to refer to the administration of substances directly to the vein i.e. via a drip.

Invasive [ɪnˈveɪsɪv] In oncology, invasive refers to a type of neoplasm which invades and spreads to other tissue. It can also refer to a type of medical procedure that involves surgical incision.

Irritable bowel syndrome (IBS) [ˈɪrɪtəbl ˈbaʊəl ˈsɪndrəʊm] A condition of the gastrointestinal tract that has symptoms including diarrhea or constipation (or both) and bloating without any obvious pathological cause. Not to be confused with Inflammatory Bowel Disease.

Ischemia [ɪˈskiːmiə] A local restriction or blockage of blood flow, which is usually caused by the constriction of the blood vessels.

Jaundice ['dʒɔːndɪs] A yellowing of the skin, sclerae of the eyes and deep tissue due to an excess of bilirubin in the blood. It can indicate the presence of liver disease or can arise in neonates because immature liver function.

K

Kaposi sarcoma (KS) [kə͵pəʊsiz sɑːˈkəʊmə] A
malignant cancer that occurs in the skin and lymph
nodes. It is most common in men over 60 years of
age and in patients infected with human herpes
virus 8, common in AIDS patients. It presents as
skin lesions with dark plaques and nodules.

Kegel exercise [ˈkeɪ gəl ˈeksəsaɪz] The contraction
and relaxation of the pelvic floor muscles to treat
urinary incontinence and for the preparation or
recovery of the pelvic floor after natural childbirth.

Keloid [ˈki lɔɪd] A nodular area of hyperplastic scar
tissue found in the subcutaneous tissue and dermis.
Keloids usually form following trauma or surgery.

Ketamine [ˈkiːtəmiːn] An anesthetic drug that
causes relaxation of the skeletal muscle, analgesia
and increased activity of the sympathetic system. It
is sometimes abused for its ability to produce
hallucination.

L

Labile ['leɪ bəl] Adaptable or easily changed. It can be used in reference to mood states or chemical property of a substance.

Labor ['leɪbə(r)] The process of giving birth or expelling a fetus and placenta from the uterus. The first stage consists of uterine contractions and cervical dilation, the second stage includes the complete cervical dilation and expulsion of the infant and the third stage in which the placenta and fetal membranes are expelled.

Lactobacillus [ˌlæktəʊbəˈsɪləs] A genus of gram-positive anaerobic bacteria found in dairy products, sewage, fermented beverages and pickles as well as naturally in the mount and GIT. They more often provide protection of pathogenic bacteria than are pathogenic themselves.

Ladder splint ['lædə(r) splɪnt] A device used for immobilizing body parts; a ladder splint is flexible and made up of two parallel wires with finer wires crossing between them.

Lamaze method [ləˈmɑz ˈmeθəd] A technique used to prepare a woman psychologically for childbirth to reduce the pains associated with labor.

Lance [lɑːns] To cut open using a lancet, which is a short, double-edged bladed surgical knife. Typically to lance refers to the opening of a boil or abscess to release pus.

Lanugo [lə'nu goʊ] The fine layer of very soft hair that covers a fetus. It appears in the fourth month of gestation and normally mostly falls off by full term.

Latency ['leɪtənsi] Having a late onset, or when there is a period of time between a stimulus and response.

Lateral ['lætərəl] On the side of an organism, either left of right. It is an anatomical term of location.

Lesion ['liːʒn] A general term for an injury or tissue damaged by disease or injury.

Let-down reflex [let daʊn 'riːfleks] Also called the milk-ejection reflex; it is the release of milk from the breast tissue resulting from the stimulation of the nipple, as when a baby suckles.

Lethal ['liːθl] Relating to or causing death. It is usually used to describe the causal agent of death, such as a dose of medication.

Licensed practical nurse (LPN) ['laɪsnst 'præktɪkl nɜːs] Also called a licensed vocational nurse, an LPN is a nurse who has graduated from a recognized course in nursing and is licensed by the state authority to practice as a nurse.

Ligament ['lɪgəmənt] A type of fibrous connective tissue which connects two or more bones or other structures, appearing as a band. Not to be confused with tendons, which connect bone to muscle.

Linea alba [lɑ 'li nɛ ɑ 'al bə] A fibrous band of connective tissue that runs vertically down the middle of the length of the abdominal wall. It is attachment point of the oblique and transverse abdominal muscles.

Linea nigra [lɑ ˈli nɛ ɑ ˈnɪgr ə] The term used to describe the linea alba during pregnancy when it becomes pigmented and often clearly visible.

Listeria [lɪˈstɪəriə] A genus of gram-positive, aerobic bacilli bacteria which causes listeriosis. It normally affects ruminants but outbreaks in humans do occur as a result of infected food sources.

Livebirth [ˈlaɪv bɜːθ] The birth of a neonate who shows evidence of life (breathing, beating of the heart, voluntary muscular movement) after being born.

Local [ˈləʊkl] Local refers to something being in the immediate area or close by. Local anesthetics numb only a small area; localized infections only affect a contained area. It is used in contrast to regional and general.

Lumbago [lʌmˈbeɪgəʊ] A general term for pain in the mid to lower back without reference to its cause.

Lumbar [ˈlʌmbə(r)] In anatomy, lumbar refers to the region between the diaphragm and the pelvis.

Lupus [ˈluːpəs] Also referred to as Systemic lupus erythematosus, lupus is an autoimmune condition where the body's immune system attacks the connective tissue in any part of the body.

Lymph [lımf] A clear fluid which is collected from interstitial spaces and flows though the lymphatic system (vessels and nodes) to a point where it is added to the venous blood. Lymph carries infectious agents and other substances to be excreted or killed by the immune system.

M

Magnetic resonance imaging (MRI) [ˌem ɑːr ˈaɪ] A type of radiologic imaging used for making diagnoses using nuclear magnetic resonance technology. It is able to create detailed images of internal structures, with especially good contrast between different soft tissues.

Malaise [məˈleɪz] A general feeling of not being well, being uncomfortable, not "feeling right". It is often a first sign of the development of a more serious condition but it may resolve itself without progression.

Malignant [məˈlɪgnənt] In oncology, malignant refers to neoplasms which are locally invasive and which have rapid metastasis.

Managed care [ˈmænɪdʒd keə(r)] A contract whereby a third party who pays for medical bills (such as an insurer) mediates between the medical professionals and the patients to negotiate fees and oversee treatment choices.

Manometer [ˈmænəʊmiːtə(r)] An instrument that measures the pressure exerted by a fluid or the difference in pressure between two fluids.

Martin bandage [ˈmɑr tn ˈbændɪdʒ] A type of rubber bandage that is used to compress parts of limbs in the treatment of varicose veins or ulcers.

Mastectomy [mæˈstektəmi] The surgical excision of the breast (partial or complete), normally indicated when there is an aggressive malignant neoplasm present but is also done prophylactically in patients who are at very high risk for breast cancer.

Mastitis [mæˈstaɪtɪs] Inflammation of the breast tissue. It is frequently due to bacterial infection and common during lactation.

Maternity hospital [məˈtɜːnəti ˈhɒspɪtl] A hospital that treats pregnant women and those giving birth.

Maximal dose [ˈmæksɪml dəʊs] The largest quantity of a drug that can be administered safely to an adult.

Maximum permissible dose (MPD) [ˈmæksɪməm pəˈmɪsəbl dəʊs] The largest dose of radiation that can be administered without causing harm to the body at a detectable level. It is given for those who are exposed acutely and chronically and it differs for individuals depending on their occupational or therapeutic exposure.

Meconium [ˈmeɪkəʊniəm] The first stool that an infant passes consisting of the cells, mucus and bile that the fetus swallowed in uterus. If passed whilst still in utero, meconium can be aspirated causing a medical emergency in the infant.

Medical examiner (ME) [ˈmedɪkl ɪgˈzæmɪnə(r)] A medical professional who examines a patient and produces a report on their physical condition to the party who requested the examination. It can also refer to the medical professional who investigates deaths from unnatural causes.

Medical record ['medɪkl 'rekɔːd] A document chronicling the treatment given to a patient, including examinations, clinical findings, diagnoses, medical therapies and procedures and related information.

Medical-Surgical Nursing ['medɪkl 'sɜːdʒɪkl 'nɜːsɪŋ] A field of nursing in which Registered Nurses work in the medical-surgical unit of a hospital. This unit deals with patients, pre- and post-surgery and pharmaceutical treatment for their illness.

Melanoma [ˌmeləˈnəʊmə] A malignant neoplasm of the cells of the skin and eyes that form melanin. They are often invasive and are especially associated with extended exposure to the sun over a lifetime.

Membrane ['membreɪn] A thin sheet of tissue which covers a part of the body or cavity, acts as a septum or connects two structures.

Meningitis [ˌmenɪnˈdʒaɪtɪs] A life-threatening inflammation of the membranes surrounding the brain and/or spinal cord, called the meninges. It is normally the result of infection by a virus or bacteria.

Mesentery ['mɛs ən ˌtɛr i] The layer and fold of the peritoneum that is attached to the abdominal wall and suspends the small intestines.

MeSH [meʃ] An abbreviation for "Medical Subject Headings", it is a controlled vocabulary for journal articles and books in the life sciences. It is maintained by the United States National Library of Medicine.

Metaplasia [mə'tæ'pleɪ ʒə] The change in cell type from one differentiated type to another. It is part of the normal development of the cell or stimulated by an external source.

Microdermabrasion [ˌmaɪkrəuˌdɜːmə'breɪʒən] A technique used to improve the appearance of the skin. It uses mechanical abrasion but is very superficial and does not strip the skin of the epithelium.

Micrometer [maɪ'krɒmɪtə(r)] A unit of measurement which is one millionth of a meter (a micron) or a device which is used under the microscope to accurately measure very small objects.

Microscope ['maɪkrəskəʊp] An instrument that allows for the visualization of microscopic objects by using a series of magnifying glasses.

Midwife ['mɪdwaɪf] A health care professional, commonly a nurse, who is trained in obstetrics and childcare and who has a major role in childbirth.

Mini-Mental State Examination (MMSE) ['mɪni 'mentl steɪt ɪɡˌzæmɪ'neɪʃn] An assessment tool to evaluate the cognitive function or mental abilities of a patient. It can be repeated to assess the progress of a patient's condition or treatment.

Minor operation ['maɪnə(r) ˌɒpə'reɪʃn] A surgical procedure that does not involve any of the vital organs and does not pose a threat to the life of the patient in itself, although complications and drug reactions can be fatal.

MMR [ˌem em ˈɑː(r)] An abbreviation for the vaccine against measles, mumps and rubella, which is commonly given to infants.

MOC [ˌem ˈəʊ siː] An abbreviation for the "Medical Officer on Call".

MOD [ˌem əʊ ˈdiː] An abbreviation used for the "Medical Officer of the Day" meaning the Doctor who is working that day.

Monoamine oxidase inhibitor (MAOI) [em eɪ əʊ aɪ] A class of antidepressants that acts by inhibiting monoamine oxidase A and increasing the levels of monoamine neurotransmitters. They are normally only prescribed when first line treatments fail.

Morbid obesity [ˈmɔːbɪd əʊˈbiːsəti] A condition characterized by excessive body weight to the extent that normal activity is affected or excessive body weight that causes a pathological condition.

Morbidity rate [mɔːˈbɪdəti reɪt] The proportion of people who die of a particular disease in a given population and in a given time period.

Morgue [mɔːg] A unit of a hospital or other facility that houses dead bodies before identification, autopsy or before they are buried or cremated.

Morphine [ˈmɔːfiːn] An alkaloid of opium that acts as a potent analgesic. Repeated use can lead to tolerance and dependence. It is commonly used for managing pain in the terminally ill or in patients with extreme levels of pain.

Mortality rate [mɔːˈtæləti reɪt] Also called the death rate, it is an estimate of the proportion of people who die in a given population calculated over a given period.

Motility test [moʊˈtɪl ɪ ti test] A test using a microscope to assess if sperm or a microorganism on a soft agar medium is motile.

Mucus [ˈmjuːkəs] The thick clear secretion of the mucous membranes. It is made up of epithelial cells, leukocytes, mucin and other solutes in water.

Murmur [ˈmɜːmə(r)] In cardiology, a murmur refers to a heart condition in which there are audible sounds (with a stethoscope) not made by the normal beating of the heart. It is usually due to leaking heart valves such that there is turbulence in the flow of blood through the heart.

MVA [em viː eɪ] An abbreviation for motor vehicle accident.

Mydriatic [ˌmɪd riˈæt ɪk] A substance or state that causes mydriasis, or dilation of the pupil in the eye.

Myoglobin (Mb, MbCO, MbO) [maɪˈəʊˈgləʊbɪn] The protein that carries and stores oxygen in the muscle. It is similar to hemoglobin but has only one heme molecule and one subunit.

Myopathy [maɪɒpəθi] A disease of the muscle tissue, especially skeletal muscle, and not caused by neural disorders.

Myopia [maɪˈəʊpiə] Also called short or near sightedness, myopia is a condition of the eye whereby only light from short distances focus on the retina.

N

NANDA [nændə] Also referred to as NANDA International, it was previously known as and stands for the North American Nursing Diagnosis Association. It is an organization that has standardized nursing terminology.

Narcosis [nɑːˈkəʊsɪs] The reversible depression of neural activity produced by a drug or chemical agent. It is distinguished from anesthesia as a stupor.

Nausea [ˈnɔːziə] The urge to vomit which manifests as an uneasiness in the upper stomach.

NCLEX [en siː el iː eks] An abbreviation for the National Council Licensure Examination. It is the recognized exam nurses in the United States take to become licensed to practice. There are two types of examinations, one for registered nurses (NCLEX-RN) and one for practical nurses (NCLEX-PN). They are created by the National Council of State Boards of Nursing, Inc.

Nebulizer [ˈnebjəlaɪzər] A medical device which creates an aerosol from liquid medication for inhalation into the respiratory tract.

Necrosis [neˈkrəʊsɪs] The death of a cell or cells caused pathologically. It causes irreversible damage to tissue and organs and can arise from a number of causes.

Needle aspiration [ˈniːdl ˌæspəˈreɪʃn] Also called Fine Needle Aspiration (FNA), it is a type of biopsy where a sample is taken using a hypodermic needle. The cells that are extracted are then examined under a microscope for abnormality. It is normally used to biopsy tissue just below the skin.

Needle-holder ['niːdl 'həʊldə(r)] Also referred to as needle forceps, it is the surgical, hand-held instrument used for holding the needle during suturing.

Neonatal [ˌniːəʊ'neɪtl] Pertaining to neonates or infants. It can describe a hospital unit, pathological state or other objects to do with very young babies.

Neoplasm ['ni ə‚plæz əm] A mass of abnormal tissue that grows faster than normal and lacks structure. It can be benign as in the case of a tumor, or malignant in the case of a cancer.

Neuroglia [nʊ'rɒg li ə] The parts of the central and peripheral nervous system that are not made up of neural cells.

Neuroma ['njʊərəʊmə] A tumor or growth on a nerve, which can be malignant or benign and can originate from any nerve tissue. It can also refer to swellings of nerves due to physical trauma.

Neurotoxin [ˌnjʊərəʊ'tɒksɪn] A toxin that acts on the nervous tissue. Many types of animal venom are neurotoxic.

Neurotransmitter ['njʊərəʊtrænzmɪtə(r)] A chemical that transmits a signal from a presynaptic cell across a synapse to another cell which it stimulates or inhibits.

NHS [ˌen eɪtʃ ˈes] An abbreviation for the National Health Service, which is the state health provision facility in the United Kingdom.

Nitrous oxide [ˌnaɪtrəs ˈɒksaɪd] A gas commonly inhaled as a fast acting analgesic for performing surgical procedures and which can rapidly be reversed as well as being nontoxic. Also called laughing gas.

Nonsteroidal anti-inflammatory drugs (NSAIDs) [nɒnˈsterɔɪdl ˈænti ɪnˈflæmətri drʌgz] A group of drugs that are, as the name suggests, anti-inflammatory and not steroids. They are often also antipyretics and analgesics and include aspirin and ibuprofen.

Norepinephrine (NE) [ˌnɔr ɛp əˈnɛf rɪn] A catecholamine derived from dopamine. It acts with epinephrine to produce the fight or flight response. It increases blood pressure through its action as a vasoconstrictor. It binds adrenergic receptors.

Nurse [nɜːs] To nurse can mean to breast-feed or to provide health care for the sick, but as a noun it describes a person who is trained in the science of nursing. Nursing is concerned with the diagnosis and treatment of medical conditions.

Nurse practitioner (NP) [nɜːs prækˈtɪʃənə(r)] A nurse practitioner is a registered nurse (an advanced practice nurse) with some advanced education in a specific field of nursing, usually a master's degree.

Nurse-client relationship [nɜːs ˈklaɪənt rɪˈleɪʃnʃɪp] The defined, interpersonal relationship that describes nurse-client interactions.

Nurse-led clinic [nɜːs led ˈklɪnɪk] A nurse-led clinic is any clinic (especially an outpatient clinic) that is managed and led by a registered nurse or nurse practitioner.

Nursing audit [ˈnɜːsɪŋ ˈɔːdɪt] The procedure used to monitor and evaluate the quality of nursing in a hospital or other facility.

Nursing care plan [ˈnɜːsɪŋ keə(r) plæn] A nursing care plan is an action plan that describes the nursing care which will be provided to a patient (this could be an individual or a family or whole community).

Nursing diagnosis [ˈnɜːsɪŋ ˌdaɪəgˈnəʊsɪs] The nursing diagnosis is a facet of the nursing process. It is the clinical decision or judgment about the state and nature of a patient's condition in terms of actual or potential health problems. It is based on information that is acquired during a nursing assessment.

Nursing Minimum Data Set (NMDS) [ˈnɜːsɪŋ ˈmɪnɪməm ˈdeɪtə set] A standardized classification system for describing nursing data. It allows for the comparison of nursing data across populations, in different clinical settings and over time.

Nursing Outcomes Classification (NOC) [ˈnɜːsɪŋ ˈaʊtkʌmz ˌklæsɪfɪˈkeɪʃn] A classification system that defines terminology used to describe possible patient outcomes, which result from the intervention of nurses.

Nursing process [ˈnɜːsɪŋ ˈprəʊses] The process of client-centered, goal-oriented health care provided by nurses to patients in line with scientific nursing theory.

Nursing theory [ˈnɜːsɪŋ ˈθɪəri] Nursing theory is the body of knowledge that is used to define and understand the nursing process and practices.

O

Oblique bandage [əˈbliːk ˈbændɪdʒ] A bandage that is applied in successive oblique turns up or down a limb.

Obstetrics (OB) [əbˈstetrɪks] The specialized branch of medicine that deals with the childbirth.

Occlude [əˈkluːd] To enclose or cut off. It often refers to vascular occlusion where a blood vessel is blocked, either artificially and intentionally or by some pathological or traumatic process.

Occupational Health Nursing [ˌɒkjuˈpeɪʃənl helθ ˈnɜːsɪŋ] Occupational and Environmental Health Nursing is a branch of nursing that deals with the health and safety of employees, especially when their employment is associated with some form of occupational or environmental hazard.

Off-label [ɒf ˈleɪbl] The use of a licensed drug for a purpose for which it was not approved for by the regulatory body that licensed it (such as the FDA).

Ointment [ˈɔɪntmənt] Ointments are semisolid substances containing pharmaceutical drugs, which are intended for external use. They use different bases (oil or water based) depending on the medicine they carry and their intended use.

Oncology [ɒŋˈkɒlədʒi] The study of neoplasms, including their causes, characteristics and treatment.

Operating Room Nursing ['ɒpəreɪtɪŋ ruːm 'nɜːsɪŋ]
The field of nursing in which Registered Nurses
work in the operating room during surgical
procedures. They can be scrub nurses, RN First
Assistant nurses or circulating nurses.

Ophthalmology [ˌɒfθæl'mɒlədʒi] The specialized
field of medicine which deals with diseases and
refractive problems of the eye.

Opportunistic pathogen [ˌɒpətjuː'nɪstɪk 'pæθədʒən]
Any disease causing agent (normally microbial)
which causes disease when the host has a
compromised immune system resulting from
another disease or drug.

Optic ['ɒptɪk] Optic refers to anything pertaining to
the eye or vision, such as the optic nerve, which
transmits signals from the eye to the brain.

Optimum dose ['ɒptɪməm dəʊs] The dose of
medication or radiation that produces the intended
effect with the minimal amount of adverse effects or
side effects.

Oral ['ɔːrəl] Oral refers to the mouth, such as per
oral, meaning to take by the mouth.

Orderly ['ɔːdəli] A hospital attendant, such as a
nurse or assistant, who assists the nurses and
doctors in caring for patients.

Organic disease [ɔː'gænɪk dɪ'ziːz] A disease that
causes some anatomical change in tissues or organs
of the body.

Orifice ['ɒrɪfɪs] An aperture or opening, often used to describe the body cavities which open to the exterior.

Orthopedics [ˌɔːθəˈpiːdɪks] A division of medicine which deals with the prevention and treatment of skeletal deformities.

Orthotics [ˌɔːθɒtɪks] The medical field that deals with creating and fitting orthoses or orthopedic devices that correct functional problems of the limbs and torso.

Osteopathy [ˌɒstiˈɒpəθi] The disease of bones or study of diseases of the musculoskeletal system.

Osteotome ['ɒstiətəʊm] An instrument used for cutting bone, especially for dental implants.

Otic [əʊtɪk] Otic refers to structures and processes pertaining to hearing and the ear.

Over-the-counter (OTC) drug ['əʊvə(r) ðə ˈkaʊntə(r) drʌg] Medicine that can be sold directly to the public without a prescription written by a health care professional. The classification of drugs for sale OTC is normally done by a governing body such as the FDA.

Oxytocin (OXT) [ˌɒksɪtəʊsɪn] A hormone, similar in structure to vasopressin, which causes contractions of the uterine muscles during labor and promotes the production and release of milk during lactation. It is also used to artificially induce labor.

P

p.c [piː siː] An abbreviation for "post cibum," meaning after meals. It is used as an instruction for administering prescribed medication.

p.o [piːəʊ] An abbreviation for "per os," meaning by mouth, or orally. It is used as an instruction for administering prescribed medication.

Package insert [ˈpækɪdʒ ɪnˈsɜːt] The printed document which normally accompanies any prescribed medicine and which contains the legal pharmacological information pertaining to the drug including active ingredients, dosage, indications and contraindications.

Packed cell volume [pækt sel ˈvɒljuːm] The volume of blood that is made up of cells, which is measured after a sample has been subjected to centrifugal forces to separate the cells from the plasma.

Palliative treatment [ˈpæliətɪv ˈtriːtmənt] The care and treatment aimed at alleviating symptoms or disease of injury without curing it.

Pallor [ˈpælə(r)] Pallor refers to a paleness in the skin or mucous membranes, normally resulting from anemia.

Palsy [ˈpɔːlzi] Palsy is another name for paralysis of a body part in which there is a loss of sensation and motor control.

Papilloma [ˌpæpɪˈləʊmə] An epithelial tumor that protrudes fror the surrounding skin tissue. It is a benign neoplasm.

Papule [ˈpæp yul] A small solid area of the skin which is elevated from the surrounding tissue.

Paracetamol [ˌpærəˈsiːtəmɒl] Paracetamol is also known as acetaminophen and is a common analgesic and antipyretic sold over the counter.

part. aeq. [pɑːt ˈiːkw] An abbreviation for the Latin term "partes aequales", meaning in parts or doses. It is used as an instruction for administering prescribed medicines.

part. vic. [pɑːt ˈvɪk] An abbreviation for the Latin term "partes vicibus", meaning in divided doses. It is used as an instruction for administering prescribed medicines.

Patch test [pætʃ test] A test to determine the skin sensitivity to a substance. It involves the application of the substance to a small area of skin and observing any changes over the subsequent 48 hours.

Pathogenic [ˈpæθəˈdʒenɪk] The characteristic of causing disease. It is used, for example, to distinguish between bacteria that cause disease (pathogenic) and those that do not.

Pathology [pəˈθɒlədʒi] A specialized field of medicine that deals with the diagnosis of disease by examining body fluids and tissue.

Patient-controlled analgesia (PCA) [ˈpeɪʃnt
kənˈtrəʊld ˌænəlˈdʒiːzɪə] A technique for
administering pain relief where the patient is able to
self-administer based on their level of pain.

Pediatrics [ˌpiːdiˈætrɪks] A division of medicine
which deals with the treatment and care of children
and their diseases.

Penicillin [ˌpenɪˈsɪlɪn] An antibiotic originally
derived from a mold. It acts especially against
gram-positive bacteria and are generally non-toxic
to humans.

Perfuse [ˈpɜːfjuːs] To force blood from an artery
into a capillary bed. The level of perfusion in the
body can be used as an indication of disease states.

Perineum [ˌperɪˈniːəm] The area between the top of
the thighs, usually defined as extending from the
coccyx to the pubis including the anus and genitalia.

Peristalsis [ˌperɪˈstælsɪs] The muscular movement
of the intestine to aid in the propulsion of ingested
substances further along the digestive tract.

Peristasis [ˌperɪˈstəsɪs] The phases during
inflammation which are characterized by a lack of
vasoconstriction.

Pessary [ˈpesəri] A type of suppository inserted into
the vagina that delivers medicine to that area.

Pharynx [ˈfærɪŋks] A structure of the respiratory
and digestive tract located at the back of the nasal

and oral cavities and above the esophagus. It is important for vocalizations.

Phlebotomy [fləˈbɒtəmi] Phlebotomy is the act of drawing blood from a vein or artery, by a phlebotomist, for subsequent diagnostic testing or for transfusion into another patient.

Photophobia [ˈfəʊtəʊˈfəʊbiə] An extreme sensitivity to light, especially of the eyes. It is a symptom of uveitis and is common with migraines.

Physiotherapy [ˌfɪziəʊˈθerəpi] Also called physical therapy, it is a medical field involved in the prevention, treatment and rehabilitation of physical disabilities resulting from disease or injury.

Pia mater [ˈpaɪ.ə ˈmeɪtər] Along with the dura mater and arachnoid, the pia mater is the innermost layer of the meninges- the membranes enclosing the spinal cord and brain.

Pica [ˈpaɪkə] An abnormal appetite for non-food or non-nutritive substances such as soil, ice and paint chips. It sometimes occurs during pregnancy and is thought to be associated with some nutritional deficiency.

Placebo [pləˈsiːbəʊ] A substance that has no active ingredient, which is given as a medicine in order to gauge the response due to believing the medicine will cure versus the response due to the action of an active ingredient.

Placenta [pləˈsentə] An organ made up of maternal and embryonic tissue, which acts as a passage of metabolic exchange between mother and fetus during pregnancy.

Plantar ['plæntə(r)] Plantar refers to the sole of the foot, as in plantar wart; a wart on the bottom of the foot.

Plaque [plæk] A general term for a differentiated patch on a body surface or an area of demyelination found in multiple sclerosis.

Platelet ['pleɪtlət] Also called thrombocytes, platelets are irregularly shaped cell fragments derived from megakaryocyte. They are important for the coagulation of blood.

Polyp ['pɒlɪp] A general term describing a tissue mass that is visible with the naked eye and which protrudes from the surface. It can be neoplastic, a site of inflammation or some other lesion.

Posterior [pɒ'stɪərɪə(r)] An anatomical term of location meaning towards the tail or back of an organism. Caudal is also used for organisms with a distinct tail. Used in contrast to anterior.

Postoperative [pəʊst 'ɒpərətɪv] The period of time following or after an operation.

Postpartum [ˌpəʊst 'pɑːtəm] Post partum means after childbirth and relates to the period of time following parturition, as well as conditions that arise during that period.

Preanesthetic [priː ˌænəs'θetɪk] Preanesthetic means before anesthesia but normally refers to the medication administered prior to an anesthetic and which act as a sedative or can act synergistically with the anesthetic.

Pressure dressing ['preʃə(r) 'dresɪŋ] A dressing that exerts pressure on the area that is dressed such that fluid cannot collect in the underlying tissue.

Preventive medicine [prɪ'ventɪv 'medɪsn] The branch of medicine which deals with the prevention of disease by understanding how it originates, how it progresses and who it affects.

Primary care provider ['praɪməri keə(r) prə'vaɪdə(r)] The primary care provider refers to the health care professional who is responsible for dealing with the majority a patient's health care needs.

Private duty nurse ['praɪvət 'djuːti nɜːs] A nurse that is hired in their personal capacity by a client or patient and who does not work for a hospital or other facility.

Prognosis [prɒg'nəʊsɪs] A prediction of the probable outcome of a disease or injury.

Progressive [prə'gresɪv] When describing a course of a disease, progressive normally means the disease advances on an unfavorable path.

Prophylaxis [ˌprəʊ fə'læk sɪs] The prevention of a disease or treatment that prevents the development of a disease, such as a vaccine.

Propofol [prə'pəʊ'fɒl] A hypnotic drug which is quick and short acting. It is used for inducing and maintaining general anesthesia or as a sedative.

Prosthesis [prɒs'θiːsɪs] A device which acts as a substitute for a missing or damaged body part.

Protocol ['prəʊtəkɒl] A specific detailed plan for a study, procedure or therapeutic regimen.

Pruritus [prʊ'raɪtəs] A general term for the sensation of itching that produces a reflex to scratch.

Psoriasis [sə'raɪəsɪs] An inherited autoimmune disease of the skin, which can be characterized by maculopapules and lesions on the joints as well as the scalp and trunk.

Psychiatric Nursing [ˌsaɪki'ætrɪk 'nɜːsɪŋ] A branch of nursing that cares for and promotes the health of psychiatric patients. It can include counseling, case management, administering treatment and health education.

Public health nurse (PHN) ['pʌblɪk helθ nɜːs] Also called a community health or community nurse, a public health nurse provides nursing care to patients in a community, usually as part of a state or regional government health department initiative.

Public Health Service (PHS) ['pʌblɪk helθ 'sɜːvɪs] Also called the United States Public Health Service (USPHS), it is a bureau of the Department of Health and Human Services.

Purgative [ˈpɜːgətɪv] An agent that is administered to evacuate the bowels.

Pus [pʌs] A thick fluid that accumulates at sites of infection or foreign bodies. It is yellow-white in color and is composed of white blood cells, liquefied tissue and cell debris.

Q

q.d. [kjuː diː] An abbreviation for "quaque die," meaning once a day. It is used as an instruction for administering prescribed medication.

q.i.d. [kjuː aɪ diː] An abbreviation for "quater in die," meaning four times a day. It is used as an instruction for administering prescribed medication.

Quot. op. sit. [kwoʊt iz ˈoʊ pəs sɪt] An abbreviation for the Latin term "Quoties Opus Sit" meaning "as often as necessary". It is used as an instruction for the administration of prescribed medicine or treatments.

R

Radiation therapy [ˌreɪdiˈeɪʃn ˈθerəpi] The therapeutic use of ionizing radiation to control the growth of malignant cells. It can be curative, adjuvant or palliative.

Random sample [ˈrændəm ˈsɑːmpl] The selection of a small subset of people, objects or substances on the basis of chance such that each member or item in the set have equal chance of being selected.

Randomized controlled trial (RCT) [ˈrændəmaɪzd kənˈtrəʊld ˈtraɪəl] In epidemiology, it is an experiment where members of a population are randomly assigned into either experimental or control groups to receive or not receive (respectively) a treatment that the study is testing.

Red blood cell [red blʌd sel] Also called erythrocytes, they are the major cell type found in blood. They contain hemoglobin, which binds oxygen, providing the body with a transport system to get oxygen all through the body.

Reflex [ˈriːfleks] A reflex is an involuntary, instantaneous response of the neuromuscular system to a stimulus, for example the knee-jerk reflex response.

Regimen [ˈredʒɪmən] A regulated course for a medical treatment, not to be confused with a regime.

Registered nurse (RN) ['redʒɪstə(r)d nɜːs] A nurse
who has graduated from a recognized nurse training
program and been licensed and registered by the
state to practice as a nurse.

Registered Nurse First Assistant nurses (RNFA)
['redʒɪstə(r)d nɜːs fɜːst əˈsɪstənt] A RNFA is a
registered nurse who deals with the entire
perioperative care process and who has
perioperative nursing certification (CNOR).

Regurgitate [rɪˈgɜːdʒɪteɪt] The action of expelling
the contents of the stomach through the mouth in
small quantities.

Remission [rɪˈmɪʃn] A decrease, disappearance or
abatement in the symptoms or severity of symptoms
of a disease or condition.

Resection [rɪˈsekʃn] A surgical excision which aims
to remove a structure or part of a structure.

Resident ['rezɪdənt] Previously referring to a doctor
who resided at a hospital, a resident is a doctor who
is associated with a hospital for the purpose of
clinical training.

Respirator ['respəreɪtə(r)] A medical appliance that
provides artificial respiration when a patient stops
breathing; in the case of respiratory failure.

Retrograde ['retrəgreɪd] In disease, retrograde
implies degeneration and a reversal of the normal
progression of biological processes.

Rh factor ['riːsəs fæktə(r)] Also known as Rhesus type, the Rh factor is an additional blood type classifier to ABO. People can be Rh positive or negative and opposite signs are not compatible for transfusions.

Rosacea [rou'zeɪʃi.ə] A vascular condition affecting the nose and upper cheeks, characterized by persistent erythema and follicular dilation.

Rotavirus ['rəutəvaɪrəs] A group of RNA viruses including Rota virus which causes gastroenteritis in humans (especially infants).

S

Sacroiliac joint [ˈes aɪ dʒeɪ] The joint between the sacrum and the ilium on either side of the pelvis.

Salmonella [ˌsælməˈnelə] A gram-negative genus of bacteria which is pathogenic in humans. Members cause Typhoid fever and other food-borne diseases.

Sciatic [saɪˈætɪk] An anatomical term referring to the ischium or hip, such as the sciatic nerve and sciatica.

Sclerosis [skləˈrəʊsɪs] A hardening of soft tissue due to hyperplasia of interstitial connective tissue.

Scoliosis [ˌskəʊliˈəʊsɪs] The abnormal curvature of spinal column, usually as a result of bone deformity that develops over time.

Scrub nurse [skrʌb nɜːs] A registered nurse who has advanced training and/or experience in assisting surgeons in the operating room. The term refers to a nurse who has scrubbed their arms and hands and wears sterile clothing and gloves to assist during surgery.

Secondary infection [ˈsekəndri ɪnˈfekʃn] An infection that occurs in an individual who is already infected by another agent.

Sedation [sɪˈdeɪʃn] In medicine, sedation is the calming of a patient by the use of a pharmaceutical sedative such that agitation is reduced.

Sepsis ['sepsɪs] Systemic inflammation resulting from infection by a pathogenic organism. It most commonly includes infection of the blood, or septicemia.

Serum ['sɪərəm] In the blood, serum is the part that remains after coagulation and removal of blood cells; not to be confused with plasma.

Sexually transmitted disease (STD) ['sekʃəli træns'mɪtid dɪ'ziːz] An infectious disease that is passed from one person to another during sexual contact. Also called a venereal disease.

Sickle cell anemia ['sɪkl sel ə'niːmiə] A recessive inherited disease of the blood in which the red blood cells are crescent shaped. Homozygous individuals for the sickle cell anemia gene develop the disease and have a shortened life expectancy but those who are heterozygous have resistance to blood borne parasites such as malaria.

Sleep apnea [sliːp æp'niːə] A condition where there is an abnormal suspension of breathing, often together with waking when breathing restarts, which results in sleepiness and fatigue during the day.

Somnolence ['sɒmnələns] Sleepiness or drowsiness, which can be normal, occurring just prior to sleep, or induced by a chemical agent.

Spasm ['spæzəm] An involuntary contraction of a muscle, which has a sudden onset and can be painful.

Sphygmomanometer [ˌsfɪgmoʊməˈnɒmɪtər] A syphygmomanometer is an instrument used for measuring blood pressure. It is made up of an inflatable cuff that goes around the arm to restrict the flow of blood, and a manometer to measure the blood pressure.

Splint [splɪnt] An appliance that is used to immobilize a joint or other body part, especially during rehabilitation following injury.

Stethoscope [ˈsteθəskəʊp] An acoustic instrument for listening to the internal sounds in the body from the outside. Typically used to listen to the heart, lungs, intestines, fetus and, in combination with a sphygmomanometer, for measuring blood pressure.

Student nurse (SN) [ˈstjuːdnt nɜːs] A student who is training to become a nurse in an accredited education program.

Subacute [sʌbəˈkjuːt] A description of a condition that is more persistent than one that is acute but less so than one that is chronic.

Subclinical [sʌbˈklɪnɪkl] The presence of a disease but without observable or measurable symptoms, normally because the disease is in an early stage or because the symptoms are masked or hidden.

Subcutaneous [ˌsʌbkjuˈteɪnɪəs] Just beneath the skin. It can refer to a type of injection or incision just under the skin, or the position of a physical object such as a blood clot (hematoma).

Superior [suːˈpɪərɪə(r)] An anatomical term of location, especially in human anatomy, meaning towards the head or above; similar to anterior. It is used in contrast to inferior.

Supine [ˈsuːpaɪn] An anatomical term of position, describing when the body is lying with the face up.

Suture [ˈsuːtʃə(r)] In surgery, a suture is a long thin material used to form a seam to keep two surfaces together, as when closing a wound or surgical incision.

Systemic [sɪˈstemɪk] Relating to the whole body or a whole system. For example, systemic diseases affect multiple organs and tissue or the whole body.

T

t.i.d [tiː aɪ diː] An abbreviation for "ter in die," meaning three times a day. It is used as an instruction for administering prescribed medication.

Tachycardia [ˌtæk ɪˈkɑr di ə] A resting heart rate that is faster than that which is normal for a person at a given age.

Tay-Sachs disease [ˈteɪˈsæks dɪˈziːz] A rare autosomal recessive genetic disorder that results in degeneration from six months old and death by age four.

Tendon [ˈtendən] A fibrous band which connects muscle to bone. Not to be confused with a ligament.

Teratogenesis [təˌræt əˈdʒɛn ə sɪs] Congenital malformations of the body, also called birth defects. They usually arise during the development of the embryo or fetus.

Tetanus [ˈtetənəs] A disease resulting from infection by Clostridium tetani. It is characterized by painful contractions of the muscles caused by a neurotoxin produced by the bacteria.

The Nursing Interventions Classification (NIC) [en ˌaɪ siː] A classification system that defines the terminology used for the typical activities that nurses perform.

Thrombosis [θrɒmˈbəʊsɪs] A blood clot in a blood vessel that can block the flow of blood. It can develop as a result of injury.

Tibia [ˈtɪbiə] One of the long bones of the leg, which articulates with the femur and the fibula and talus. It is medial to the fibula and larger in size.

Tonic [ˈtɒnɪk] In a medical context, tonic refers to a state of prolonged muscle contraction or continuous, repetitive action.

Topical anesthesia [ˈtɒpɪkl ˌænəsˈθiːʒə] The loss of sensation on the surface of the skin or a mucous membrane as a result of applying a local anesthetic ointment or solution.

Tourniquet [ˈtʊənɪkeɪ] A tool used to stop the flow of blood to and from a limb or extremity by applying pressure equally around the circumference of that limb or extremity.

Triage [ˈtriːɑːʒ] An approach used especially in emergency rooms to treat patients in order according to the seriousness of their injuries or illness such that critically ill patients are treated before patients with less serious conditions.

Triple screen [ˈtrɪpl skriːn] The test done on a pregnant woman's blood for alpha-fetoprotein, chorionic gonadotropin and unconjugated estrogen, which can indicate an increased risk of the fetus having a chromosomal abnormality or neural tube defect. Also called a triple screen.

Trisomy [ˈtraɪsəʊmɪ] The condition of having an extra chromosome in the somatic cells, which is 47 chromosomes in humans instead of 46. The type of trisomy is named after the chromosome that is duplicated and each is characterized by different symptoms.

U

Ulcer [ˈʌlsə(r)] A lesion of the skin or mucous
membrane which can also be called a canker sore.
They have a variety of causes but normally persist
due to inflammation and/or infection.

Urea [jʊˈriːə] The primary product of nitrogen
metabolism in humans and other mammals. It is
excreted in the urine.

Urogenital system [ˌjʊə.rəʊ ˈdʒen.ɹ.təl ˈsɪstəm] All
of the organs involved in reproduction and the
production and excretion of urine.

V

Vaccine [ˈvæksiːn] Vaccines are medical preparations used to improve the immunity of an organism against a specific disease. It is normally injected and is typically made from an inactivated, killed or partial version of the organism that causes the disease. They are generally used as a prophylactic to prevent infection.

Vascular [ˈvæskjələ(r)] Referring to the blood vessels including arteries, veins, arterioles, venules and capillaries.

Vasectomy [vəˈsektəmi] A surgical procedure to remove a segment of the vas deferens, normally done to sterilize men who do not want to father children in the future.

Vegetative state [ˈvedʒɪtətɪv steɪt] A vegetative state is one where a person is mildly aroused from a coma but not fully conscious. It results from brain damage. The state can be persistent or permanent.

Vein [veɪn] Veins are blood vessels that carry blood towards the heart. They carry de-oxygenated blood, except for the pulmonary and umbilical veins. Veins contain valves to stop blood flowing back.

Virulence [ˈvɪrələns] The degree to which an infectious organism causes disease, including how infectious it is and the severity of the disease it causes.

Vital capacity (VC) [ˈvaɪtl kəˈpæsəti] Also called the respiratory capacity, it is the maximum volume of air that can be exhaled from the lungs after the greatest possible inhalation. The total lung capacity includes the reserve volume as well.

Vital sign [ˈvaɪtl saɪn] Physiological statistics that can be taken to assess the well being of a person. It normally includes the blood pressure, body temperature, heart and respiratory rate.

W

Ward [wɔːd] A room in a hospital or other medical facility which houses patients with similar conditions or who are receiving similar treatments.

Wet compress [wet kəmˈpres] A compression bandage that is moistened with a saline or antiseptic solution that prevents the underlying tissue from drying out or becoming infected.

Whooping Cough [ˈhuːpɪŋ kɒf] The common name for pertussis, which is an acute inflammation by Bordetella pertussis. It affects the larynx, trachea and bronchi and is recognized by the whooping sound of the larynx in spasm when coughing.

X

X-ray [ˈeks reɪ] In medicine, x-rays are the use of ionizing radiation to produce images of internal structures, especially the bone and tumors. It is minimally invasive and important in the diagnosis of a range of conditions.

Z

Zoonosis [ˌzoʊ.əˈnoʊsɪs] An infectious disease that can be passed from animals to humans.

Zygote [ˈzaɪgoʊt] The diploid cell that forms when the egg fuses with the sperm at fertilization.

About Minute Help

Minute Help Press is building a library of books for people with only minutes to spare. Follow @minutehelp on Twitter to receive the latest information about free and paid publications from Minute Help Press, or visit minutehelpguides.com.

Printed in Great Britain
by Amazon

67001922R00058